BEATING

DEPRESSION

&

LIVING WITH CANCER

BEATING DEPRESSION & LIVING WITH CANCER

visit: htpps://www.createspace.com/3372021

Also by Sol Kesler

JUDGEMENT: JERUSALEM

visit: htpps://www.createspace.com/3370337

LEGEND: LOGOS

visit: htpps://www.createspace.com/3370340

ARCHITURE: PARADIGM or PARADOX?

visit: htpps://www.createspace.com/3413809

ROCKLANDS BEACH STORIES

BEATING DEPRESSION & LIVING WITH CANCER

Written In loving memory of Nora.

Who had it tougher than most.

Visit. htpps://www.foldapod.com

INTRODUCTION

This is a different kind of book. Sure, it's about beating depression and living with cancer. Cancer or any dreaded disease. But it's mainly about depression because diseases spawn depression so it's understandable the two should go together although it is not always so.

Basically, beating depression is part of a mind game which, together with those dreaded diseases, can be *managed* by one's mental approach. While medication is essential, beyond that there's still work to do. Simple, physically undemanding, mind work.

This is not a medical book for reasons you'll soon learn and, anyway, there are enough of those and they all explain that you're depressed because of certain symptoms you display. This book is different because, while cancer and depression are health things, the author is not a medical person. Far from it. I am, in fact, an architect. So I can't explain, clinically, why you're depressed. But, the medical fraternity can't either. Not entirely because, while medical science knows a lot about depression, it isn't positive on why it happens. So you don't have to be a health professional to write this kind of book which is more concerned with the effects of depression and how you handle them than the causes. To me, it's what you do about depression that counts. Living with depression and in finding a path through it, I learned how to *manage* my problems. Clinicians doesn't usually have that personal insight and, let's face it, you don't have to know how a computer works to use one. Or understand the internal combustion engine to drive a motor car. So I guess I'm qualified.

But please don't get me wrong. I have the greatest respect for, and trust in, the medical profession. They've kept my cancer at bay and me alive these past fourteen years. Thanks to them, my latest C.T. scans and blood tests show that I'm cancer free; no sign at all of any semenoma or lymphoma. Or any other bugs. Those abdomen and thorax tumours have disappeared which adds my name to a very long list of cancer survivors. I'm also a depression beater because that too has gone.

Having a "dreaded disease" (only an insurance company could have thought up that description) is a prime cause of depression. I can think of nothing else that comes remotely close because mortality plays a huge role in causing it. Which does not mean that you also have a dreaded disease if you're depressed. Not at all.

So why, you ask, is an architect writing about depression and cancer when he should be designing buildings?

I'm writing about depression and cancer because I've been involved in my mortality for a long time now and I seem to have come out on top. Which means I've learned a thing or two which qualifies me to spread the word. In today's idiom, I've walked the walk and talked the talk so I should know what I'm talking about. In a sense I'm still there but feeling a lot better about it. I learned things because I had to find a way through so many dreads and fears. In doing so, I found a direct path through the maze that is psychiatry, radiotherapy, pathology, oncology and chemotherapy. Looking back, I'd say it had a lot to do with my positive attitude. There were times in the chemo room when I shouted "chemo gives me wings!" Shouted it out loud just to keep my spirits up. To the obvious disapproval of fellow sufferers.

What about the health professionals who have treated or are treating you? How many have been where you are? And who in their right mind would want to endure anything like it? Sure they can describe the symptoms and prescribe the necessary. In doing so, they're acting from "afar". Because they have had to take a few steps back to get a wide angled view of our problem. I suppose the computer and motor car analogies apply here as well, albeit in reverse. Which in essence, is the reason why I've written this book.

I know I can help you so here's the deal. Like the professionals I've also detailed depression's symptoms. Even if I hadn't already experienced most of them I could, with impunity, list them directly from the Internet because it's all public domain stuff. But I do better than compiling a list. I tell you things you won't find on the Internet or anywhere else for that matter. In this little book, I describe, logically and in detail, how to manage your symptoms. I know you can beat depression because I have and I'm no genius.

Sure, it's been a long haul because lady luck pitched me a curve ball known as depression along with the cancer. What I thought was just a whiff of depression to make life interesting turned out to be something else. When it happened, the whiff didn't seem as perilous as young artillery lieutenant Napoleon Bonaparte's whiff of grapeshot that put down an unruly mob during the early stages of the French Revolution. So much for *liberte, egalite, fraternite.*

But enough of that. We have now come to an important moment.

If you are to proceed with this regimen, the time has come to adopt the attitude you will need to beat depression, the approach to which you will have to commit yourself if you are to live decently again with or without a dreaded disease.

Again, I repeat. Being depressed doesn't mean that you have, or will contract, a dreaded disease. The medical conditions are obviously very different. The link connecting them is emotion which can be extremely strong so your mental approach becomes critical. Because it will determine the kind of mind 'game' you'll have to play to beat depression. Don't panic. The 'game' only involves mental effort which isn't difficult to handle.

I say again, the connection between depression and a dreaded disease is emotional. Obviously, these conditions co-exist in the same body so they must be healed by the same mind. Which means you've got to get your mind right and that, in turn, suggests the need for some kind of an emotional anti-biotic; anti-depressive medication strong enough to let you live quite decently with depression. How successful you'll be depends largely on how well you apply yourself.

Here's what I've discovered about depression. Yes. In my case, "discovered" is the right word. It was, in a sense, on a voyage of discovery, that I learned about depression; a discovery nothing like Columbus's daring voyage to the east by going west. Or Vasco da Gama beating everyone to the sea route to India via the Cape of Good Hope to get at those spices. Like everyone, I started my voyage not suspecting that I was to measure fathoms of mental frustration and despair such as I could never have imagined.

But, again, enough of that. You're depressed so you should be on anti-depressive medication so you should be feeling better. Isn't that enough? No! You must do something to stabilise your gains because *you* are at risk here. If anything comes unstuck, you, dear reader, will be the fall guy. You'll have to stand and fight, or flee. That's why they call it fight or flight.

Now a soft word in your ear. Please know that, in everything you do, you are your own best expert. Simply because you are always in the firing line. No matter what learned professionals say or do, if they are wrong or if anything goes awry, you, dear reader, will pay. That's why this book urges you to get actively involved in your own recovery. Don't leave it entirely to others no matter how competent they might be. Or appear to be. I'm not suggesting that you ignore professional advice. Not at all but if aren't comfortable with something, look further. Get another, other opinions. Be sceptical because ultimately *you* must be your own judge and jury because it's in your own interest to do so.

Please don't beat yourself up about me being an architect. Sure, I might be a designer, a planner, a builder; all those things, but first and foremost, I'm a depressive and a cancer victim. Because I've been there, my professional training helped me plan my strategy. First came information gathering. Then information analysis and, finally, synthesis; the solution, much like any design. OK, so I'm not qualified to comment on the clinical does and the don'ts. I accept that without reservation because I know as much about diagnosis and prognosis as any medical man knows about construction. But I do know how I reacted to cancer and to depression. I recall the hard time I had dealing with a suddenly changed life. Stuff I learned from the medics and the data I gleaned from literature issued by the United States National Institute of Mental Health. Especially the USA because it is rumoured that half of America is on Prozac. An unfair exaggeration, I know. All because of a drug called fluoxetine. A k a Prozac. Or it's many generics.

SECTION ONE

1   ABOUT DEPRESSION

You're reading this so you already know that depression is a mental thing, a chemical imbalance in the brain. Sounds bad, I know, but it's really only got to do with stuff called serotonin and a few other brain mystery components. To simplify the whole spiel, beating depression is really an emotional mind game. You could call it a contest of wills. Sounds very intellectual and complicated which, medically, it is. But for our purposes you don't have to know much more about the human brain, to work it out.

Getting back to basics, you've long discovered there is a right way to do things and a wrong way and beating depression is no different. As far as I am concerned, my way (sounds like Sinatra!), the information I'm going to pass on to you is the right way albeit my personal answer to our problem. It includes a "knack". A secret within the secret. I've discovered there is one sure way to beat depression. To put paid to it's debilitations. And I'm prepared to put my head on a block (talk about the French Revolution!) to support my claim!

It's very simple so please don't be disillusioned when you read the next bit. When I reveal all because, by now, you're expecting some great revelation. You've imagined the mental isometrics you'll have to get into to rid yourself of the scourge. That's not so at all. What I've got to tell you is really very basic.

You're impatient. "Enough! Get to the point!"

You want to know what I'm talking about. The thing that's so easy? What is the so-called secret? O.K. I give it to you now. In upper case font.

GET YOUR MIND OCCUPIED ON OTHER THINGS AND KEEP IT THERE! BECAUSE DEPRESSION CAN'T DO A THING TO YOU WHEN YOU'RE NOT THINKING ABOUT IT.

I told you it's simple? But easy? Not always!

Well, so much for the big secret. Now for the trick, the knack.

Question: When I'm deeply depressed, how do I get into that occupied mental state and then stay there? In other words, how can I get there when I can't even think straight?

Answer: That is what depression has done to you and getting you out of there, dear reader, is what this book is about.   I'll show you how but first listen up and listen carefully.   I cannot overstress the need for professional remedial help. Conventional medicine. Traditional. Herbal? Whatever your bent.   Whatever works for you.   Anything you're comfortable with. *As long as it works.*

Again I stress that while medication will help to clear your mind, it is not the panacea.   It won't fix depression entirely.   To get there you've got to add something of yourself.   You have to work your own initiative into the equation. Because with that comes the cure. Medication is essential because it will *relieve* your depression. As long as you're on it, it will keep you going albeit in a surrealistic kind of way.   But it will give you the space you need to start thinking coherently again. And when you're in that mind set, you'll begin to build the mental springboard from which you'll launch your campaign against depression. In other words, you need the mental relief medication provides to get you out of the starting blocks and onto the track. Once there, you'll power your way to the tape.

"I'll never do it!" you plead.   "It's impossible! I don't have a mind of steel?"

Wrong! You don't need a mind of steel to become what you once were. To regain your normality. However, there's a *caveat.* A clear message. Again, it's fight or flight. Accept depression and succumb; flee. Or stay and fight and win. Fight isn't the word of choice because there's nothing rigorous about it. There are only two antagonists and they're both in your own head. They are your "normal" mind versus your "depressed" mind. Also, they're not fighting. They're just sparring in front of a mirror, facing every thought with thought. Every emotion with emotion. The action is in your cranium and it's not brutal. Just a place where mental rough and tumble happens. But know this. The one thing your brain understands best of all is itself. Which immediately puts you on the winning side because you're your own best friend. And enemy.

Again I hear your hapless cry. "I can't face it! I'm too stressed out, too unsettled! Too numbed by depression!"

That's not true at all. You can do it and I'll show you how. Goals. You have to set goals. Rationally. One at a time. I'll show you how to set each goal and how to achieve them. You'll be encouraged when you see that you're winning, that you're getting there. However, another caveat, more advice. Don't be impatient. It'll happen. But not overnight.

Ever heard of the adage, "the strong take from the weak but the clever take from the strong"? Or "if you can't be strong, be clever"? It's going to happen to you. You're going to get clever.   But I'll need your full co-operation. What I propose is effortless stuff but like everything else in life, it needs your best shot.   So the more you put into this mind game – that's how I'd like you to think of it - the more you'll get out of it.

Something else before we get going. You may think I'm too flippant about something this serious.   Relax. I'm doing it deliberately because when the chips are down you don't gain anything by being funereal. For sure, depression and a DD (dreaded disease) are not things to laugh about but it's best to lighten up when you're planning your moves. Even if it's only bravado.

In   this   book,   I've   relied   entirely   on   personal experiences so, in describing feelings, sensations and situations, I write of my own feelings, sensations and the situations in which I found myself. It's natural to write about things you know.   In my view, the best way to explain or describe depression is by bringing reality back to its abstract world. When you're there but you're not really there. I think you know what I mean. So please bear with me and, as you read, imagine yourself in the situations I describe. Do that and you'll begin to associate because we all face depression in much the same way.   We may not face the same *symptoms* but the mental attitude we need to develop is much the same.

3   WHY I GOT DEPRESSED:

For me it was the good life. Happy days lingering on the beach, swimming the cold Atlantic. Feeling the sun tingling my skin, sensing those ultra-violets and infra reds filtering into my body without worrying about it being good or bad for me? Yes! Those were really happy days, jogging, striding, walking the beachfront promenade and the lawns, feeling the grass between my toes twice a day. Early every morning and late every afternoon. All Speedo'd, barefooted and ready to roll. Yes. That's how it was. I was healthy. I was fit. I was good!

THEN, SUDDENLY, IT ALL CHANGED.

Can you beat it?

I never realised how good I'd had it. How good it had been enjoying the simple pleasures. Living clean, eating, drinking, laughing, joking. Aah! The *"joie de vivre"*.

UNTIL, SUDDENLY, IT ALL CHANGED.

Question. Will it ever be the same? Will I ever laugh, smile, sing again?

Answer. Yes. It will. Yes, you will. All is not lost. But to get back to what you were will take work, effort and patience. Determination and brainwork and a better understanding of what you're up against and what you need to do about it. How to go about handling your changed life. How to deal with your problem. Our problem, really. Yours and mine and millions like us because we're all charter members of Depressives International, the biggest club in the world.

You ask yourself why life changed but inside you suspect because you wouldn't have picked up this little book, wouldn't have glanced through it or bought it unless, deep down, you knew something was wrong. Maybe you were just feeling different. Perhaps you'd noticed a change in your metabolism which has now been pinned down to depression. There is always at least one reason why depression gets to you. Like it or not, you've developed this mental thing, this serotonin or norepineephrine (whatever) imbalance for which there are many causes. And many permutations.

My imbalance resulted from traumatic emotional stuff that became clinical. In my case, it started with cancer. I would never have believed it but it showed that however which way we look at things, we never know what the future holds. Or how the cookie is going to crumble. But that's what life is about so don't beat yourself up about it. Don't dwell on it. Accept it. David, biblical king of Israel and big-time Psalmist - I suspect he was a depressive - (also, incidentally, the best selling writer of all time), said, in Psalm 39, "Oh let me know my time, O G-d. And the number of my days. What they are and may I know when I will cease to be." We'll all cease to be but I certainly don't want to know when. Surely it's more fun our way?

Back to my story. Other things also happened to me but cancer alone was enough to bring on a bad case of depression. And anxiety. The cancer started out as an 'atypical' semenoma. Testicular cancer. Resulting in an orchydectomy (to the unitiated, a testicular procedure) followed by heavy doses of radiation. But that was only the beginning because then my wife had a stroke and died unexpectedly. So the cancer reared again but turned out to be high grade, non Hodgkins lymphoma. So much for the 'atypical' semenoma: beware the 'a' before 'typical' in any medical report. Which brought on more tests; ultrasound and CT scans and the pictures weren't good! Maybe because I forgot to smile!

But what followed was no laughing matter although I did find myself in the theatre! Bone marrow samples, pathologists, oncologists, more procedures, other surgeons, hospitals and the surgical theatres I mentioned, tongue in cheek four lines back. Radiotherapy again and then something new; chemotherapy to give the old body a charge because radiotherapy is such a bore! I mean, what's so fascinating about lying on a carbon fibre table with radiation coursing through your body at velocities approaching the speed of light? I worked out that, according to Einstein's e=mc2, if the potential energy in my body was equal to the difference in the "before and after" *reaction* mass of my body, multiplied by the speed of light, squared, it meant I'd been schlepping around a pile of energy for years. No wonder I was always bushed.

And that's only in terms of nuclear fission; energy released on Hiroshima. Nuclear fusion is something else entirely. If you're interested, fusion is the source of energy unearthed when very small bits of differing particles are fused together without the exotic release of fission's energy. Particles like water vapour and - I hope I've got this right - lithium. I must be right about lithium because lithium salts are used to treat manic or bi-polar depression!

My story is hardly told but that's all you're going to hear. You know enough to be convinced that I've earned my stripes. I've graduated and I'm entitled to my depression. It's my due. My right. My reward? Hardly. But it shows that depression isn't just having the blues. For me it was the result of severe trauma which can sometimes hit you like a ton of bricks but is usually more gradual. And, like radiotherapy, accumulative. Also, it can last a while if you let it.

The United States National Institute of Mental Health, in its NIH Publication No. 00-3561, titled "Depression", printed 2000 and upgraded 04/09/2004, states that "a depressive disorder is an illness that involves the body, mood and thoughts. It affects the way a person eats and sleeps, the way one feels about oneself and the way one thinks about things. A depressive disorder is not the same as a passing blue mood. Nor is it a sign of personal weakness. Or a condition that can be willed or wished away. People with a depressive illness cannot 'pull' themselves together' and get better. Without treatment, "symptoms can last for weeks, months or years. Appropriate treatment, however, can help most people who suffer from depression."

I've structured this book in two sections. Section One, where we are now, tells you how to face up to and handle depression in all its facets. Section Two gives you a general account of depression and anxiety; the two can go hand in glove. Together with the symptoms much of which any "seasoned" depressive will already know. I've included Section Two to inform new victims. It's got the kind of information I desperately needed when it all started for me. However, there's nothing to stop you from starting with

Section Two, if you want to get the facts first and then go "back to the beginning".

While it may sound exotic, lymphoma is not exactly a treat and, thankfully, many cancers are manageable if you catch them early. Many of us are tributes to our awareness, to the interest we take in our bodies. But mainly to the high standards of the medical profession and its professionals. Accordingly, I salute my wonderful medical team. Thank you so very much for everything. I'm still here because of you.

Beyond that, in more than a small way, I'm convinced beating depression has to do with being positive. Is that why I have coped? Is that why I'm still here, writing about it?

3

BEATING DEPESSION & DEALING WITH A DREADED DISEASE

Setting aside the causes for the moment, I consider depression and *anxiety* to be collective nouns for an amalgam of symptoms later listed.

Depression's symptoms are difficult to fathom when we think of them collectively. And that's where we go wrong because we shouldn't group them together. The Gestalt school of psychology maintains, in simple terms, that visually, the whole is more than the sum of it's parts. Which, to me, means that if we tackle the parts separately, we have a better chance of getting at the 'whole' in a more concerted way.

The other side of the coin is collectivity. In my view, collective 'anythings' are usually suspect. Collective guilt, collective conscience, etc. Whichever way you look at it, we are individuals, not collectives and that strengthens my resolve to think of depression's causes as individual influences. Sure. You suffer from depression or anxiety. Or both. But that's just a semantic something for the symptoms that rule and ruin your life. Each one of us can lay claim to some symptoms from the list that follows but we are all different, so we won't all suffer all the same symptoms all the time. And certainly not to the same extent. Depression isn't like flu or measles or malaria where things follow an established clinical pattern. And you can't notice depression in others because no-one runs a temperature or shows spots and things.

To ease the overwhelming mental burden of depression, I've stripped the signs collective down to symptom, singular. You'll find a similar symptoms list in other books on the subject. They're all invaluable because they tell you what you're up against.

Again the questions.

What brings it on? How long does it last?

Questions. Questions. Alas, too many of those and too few answers. Sorry, no clinical answers in these pages either. Just tips, words of "wisdom", of encouragement and advice. Suggestions how to go about beating the scourge. Stuff that's embedded in my mind because I've endured general depression in most of it's phases, and, strangely, I've also luxuriated in its very few but daunting revelations. Yes! There are those as well; the other side of the moon. The kind of revelation that's so bizarre you'll be gobsmacked. But more about that later.

Sure, I've wallowed, despairingly, in depression's lows. Teeth and clamped jaws stuff. Hell on earth. But it didn't last forever.   Not with correct remedial help. Psychotherapy helps tremendously so visiting a shrink or a psychologist isn't something to avoid or to be ashamed of because they're health practitioners who know what they're about. I settled for a psychiatrist on the recommendation of my GP when his treatment didn't seem to help much. The shrink put me on a stronger dose of the same anti-depressant and it worked. Which made me realise that by starting with correct treatment and by then adding the hints detailed in this booklet, you will beat depression.

Solzhenitsyn, Russian Nobel "Gulag" laureate wrote about the bad not lasting forever while the good seldom overflowed the cup. Wise words and so very true especially when they're describing depression.

I've still got a lot of humour in me. Which means I'm not a pessimist.   But certainly no philosopher or healer either. Nothing at all like Plato, Schweitzer or Freud. But I've learned certain things about depression and what I have to pass on to you should be reassuring. Like the cliched light at the end of the tunnel. Also it won't hurt to hear that the depressive cloud is not radioactive and that it does have a silver lining. My sincere wish is that one day soon you'll see that lining and reach out for it. And when you do, when you embrace it, hold on tight and never let go because it is truly a precious and wonderful thing.

Now back to the facts.

Get active and stay active. It's the best thing to do because depression can't do a thing to you when you're thinking of other things. When your mind is busy, you're already coping. Suddenly you're unaware of the problem and for those moments, you've forgotten what depression is. I repeat, the secret is getting there. The trick is staying there.

It will cheer you to know that depression sufferers have done great things. People like Lord, Sir Winston Churchill, British war leader, politician, Nobel laureate, erstwhile Boer War correspondent. Aristocrat of the House of Marlborough. Kin of John Churchill, 1st Duke of Marlborough, General and Statesman, regarded by many as one of the greatest military commanders of all time. Winston was one of us. He called his depression "the black dog on my back." Without depression, can you imagine how much more the man would have achieved? Alas, unfortunately, there is the flip side. Painter Vincent van Gogh was an epileptic who only sold one painting in his lifetime and literary Nobel Laureate, Ernest Hemingway also suffered from depression. What heights their achievements. Their creations? Above all, we must be aware of an untimely end. It is that which makes depression life threatening.

4   SYMPTOMS OF DEPRESSION

Consider the following list and decide if you're depressed. Hopefully, you won't be suffering from all of them. Perhaps only a combination or a permutation. And don't let the long list throw you.

1   Difficulty getting out of bed and starting the Day.

2   Deteriorating quality of life.

3   Where's the laughter?

4   Reduced libido.

5   Thoughts of suicide.

       (a k a What's the point of it all?)

6   Need for medication or therapy.

7   Confusion. Decision making, Concentrating, Memory lapses.

8   Severe tension and stress.

9   Pessimism: Feelings of hopelessness.

10   Disinterest in activities once enjoyed.

11   Bad "nerves", Tremours and jumpiness.

12   Unexplained physical disorders

13   Lethargy (a k a Lack of motivation & initiative).

14   Personal hygiene & appearance

15   Loss of self esteem.

16   Guilt.

17   Anxiety

5   WHAT TO DO ABOUT IT?

Some of the above symptoms can be grouped together insofar as treatment dynamics is concerned. It is interesting to note that, except for suicide, the list seems innocuous. Don't believe it. All are extremely debilitating. I've already stated that a depressive usually suffers from a number of symptoms simultaneously without displaying even a clue. It's not as if you've had an operation and have something to show for it. Like a scar or a wound. Or the crutches I was supposed to use after my sartorius muscle surgery.

And there's a touch of humour in that story as well. So let me tell you about it. In the ward, after surgery on my sartorius muscle; the lymphoma had spread, this character loomed suddenly at my bedside.

Surprised, I asked, "Who are you?" I was more surprised when he smiled.

"I'm your physiotherapist."

"Haven't got one," I retorted. "And anyway, what for?"

An audible sigh; he'd been there before. "I'm here to teach you how to walk again."

"Teach me?" I asked incredulously. "To walk?"

"Surgeon says you need crutches."

"Crutches? Nonsense! I walk to the bathroom on my own. Let me show you."

And I did.

"You need crutches," he insisted, producing aluminium things as tall as my elbows. "I'll show you how to use them. And give you a few exercises so you'll learn how to walk. Even up and down the stairs."

So I learned what to do with the crutches on the level and up and down the stairs but I never used them. In or out of hospital. However, my grandkids loved them, played with them for weeks. Used to shoot at things or used them as pointers. The question is, did loss of part of my sartorius muscle theoretically render me disabled? I have often wondered whether I had suddenly graduated, was now permitted to use parking spaces reserved for physically challenged folk? I suppose I would have had I relied upon the crutches. But I had never used them and it wasn't as if I was in a wheelchair or anything. All I showed was something approaching a limp and not too much of that either.

But wasn't it enough? After all, I had lost something. So where was the recognition? The reward? Emotionally and physically, I'd been through the radiology, surgery, pathology, oncology mill. In that order. And I had lost something in the suffering but then I had also lost my appendix aeons back and had a remodeled prostrate to boot. So I never took the thought further and I've never parked in those choice spaces. Although I have been tempted.

6 DEALING WITH THE SYMPTOMS

ANALYSIS.

This is the starter tip, the *numero uno.* So sit yourself down and study the full list again and then decide which of them belong to you; those you thumbed down on depression's highway or those you inherited along the genetics trail. Tick any item even if you only *suspect* it might be you. There is bound to be more than one so find some paper and list them. Hopefully the fewer the better but don't be alarmed if there are several. Be true to yourself because it's important.

When you've written them down, think about each one carefully and then accept the facts. If you're depressed, admit it out loud to yourself and to those close to you. Don't be ashamed. Depression is not a weakness. It's an illness like any other, less than some but worse than most. This is important because acceptance is the first step to recovery. Don't be too macho or macha (?). Don't shrug anything off because you'll be fooling yourself and that won't help. Be honest. Acknowledge the symptoms and you're on your way. Soon you'll be able to deal with them because now, for the first time, you know *and accept* what you're up against.

That's the first step established. Now here's how you advance. Step by step.

SYMPTOM #1

DIFFICULTY GETTING OUT OF BED AND STARTING THE DAY.

Bed. Womb. Haven. Whatever you wish to call it. It's the place where you best like to hide, where you best like to be. Sorry. You've got to get out of there! You're in trouble because depression thrives under those conditions; like flowers under glass or rabbits in a warren. What? You can't get up? Oh yes, you can. Here's how to condition your mind.

Set yourself a time to get out of bed in the mornings. Prepare your mind the night before. Decide on a "get up" time before you fall asleep, when there's no pressure. Then, in the morning when you're awake, use the TV, the radio or the alarm clock. Whatever and tell yourself you'll get out of bed after the morning news or the weather report. Make as if there is an urgent, pressing need. Like desperately needing the bathroom which will get you up quick enough so do the same now. Throw off the covers when that "dreaded" moment arrives. Then it's go.

I used to wait for the weather forecast and got up the moment I heard the forecast temperatures for my city. The temperatures weren't always right and I've never heard climatologists apologise for their errors but they certainly got me up. It worked. But you must do it every morning. I mean, you're going to get up eventually so why not then and there? You've already prepared your mind so accept what you've got to do and do it! Even though you're hating yourself for even thinking about it.

Good! So you're up? Now what?

Don't get back into bed1

Start your morning routine. Everybody has one but if you don't, work one out now. It's mundane but so very important. Think about what you're going to do when you're up. Go to the bathroom, boil the kettle, make tea. Or coffee? Instant or perked? Shave. Brush your teeth. Bath or shower then dry and dress. What colour underpants? What shirt? Short or long sleeved or T? Comb your hair. Have breakfast. You know what you've got to do so work it all out. What for breakfast? Porridge? What kind? Maybe a cereal? What? Cold milk or hot? Eggs. Boiled, scrambled, fried or poached? Or an omelette? And jam? Apricot, marmelade or strawberry? Or Marmite on toasted white or brown or whole-grain bread? There's a lot to think about so plan ahead. Before you get up you must know what you're going to do next. Decide on those silly, simple things. Like what you're going to do the moment you're on your feet even if it's only to make coffee or tea. Perhaps it's something important like saying your prayers. The same things you've been doing for years, things you've always done but never really thought about. Slip into that old familiar routine, those familiar, comfortable things because that's what you need right now.

I'm not very religious but I do pray and prayer has became a very powerful control. I benefit most from its tranquility, the warmth I feel when I'm praying. It's as if Someone is listening. Someone is reaching out to me. Someone up there is taking a personal interest in me. I feel good when I'm praying so G-d must be listening and I'm not alone. Surely He must have noticed me a long way back because I'm a fourteen year cancer survivor.

Prayer helped me get started because my morning routine slotted in very well. Or *vice versa*. If you don't have set prayers, compose your own. Think and write them down. It's such a pity that few folk compose their own prayers. That's why we have printed prayer books. When composing your personal prayers, don't worry about style and be sincere. Be yourself because you're preparing a plea, you're asking for something.   Make it a sermon to yourself. Concentrate on what you want to say or ask or declare. Let it come from the heart because you're involved with your Maker. Then as the days go by, slowly expand your prayers. Add new thoughts, those new things you've wondered about. Always praise Him before you ask for help. And always thank Him for the air you breathe, the sights you see and the sensations you experience.

Read your prayer every morning. Soon, you'll know it by heart and you'll experience a joy, a feeling of refuge, a sense of belonging that only prayer provides. When you're praying, there is a great Power beside you. Someone Who'll see you right, Who'll see you through your problems. There is a Judaic prayer: "Cast thy burden on the Lord and He will sustain thee". I believe that and I truly believe you should not only call on G-d when you need Him. Dedicate times to your Maker during the day. Acknowledge and thank Him for what He has done, is doing and shall, you pray, continue to do.

The morning routine done, get your mind working. Theorise. It's part of the therapy. When I've got the time, I think about Man and wonder why he is so curious of the great beginning. Why he seeks scientific answers to Genesis. Why he wants to uncover the "building blocks" of the universe. He wants to know what they're made of? He wants to know the meaning of life? I find it strange that the more science inquires, probes, theorises and researches, the deeper and deeper it subsides into a quagmire, a morass of the minuscule. Scientists now know more and more about less and less. Example. Once atoms were the mystery. Now it's quarks. And anti-matter. Soon, no doubt even as I write, they're discovering things more minute. Can't we see where this is going, where these discoveries are taking us? We're sinking more and more into the minuscule. Doesn't it suggest that the ever expanding infinite universe, as some claim it to be, also embraces an ever expanding, balancing minimal framework which reaches forever beyond the touch of man to an introspective infinity that counterbalances the 'extraspective' macro universe?

And I wonder why science doesn't do an about turn? To me, it suggests that in searching for proof of genesis, we should turn away from the micro and head back towards the macro, to again research the philosophical, the metaphysical, the ontological with the same zest that science probed the minuscule? Shouldn't we turn, perhaps, to a priori answers, to questions unsolved by scientific observation, analysis or experiment. In other words, shouldn't we turn back to our oldest texts, the oldest writings and reconsider those answers we derided as being unscientific. Isn't it weird that man has leaped into space, has explored, has reveled in walkabouts on the moon, has sent probes into the vast dark unknown, has photographed planets, has even landed his machines only to abandon them there as monuments to his technological prowess? So he proved that the moon isn't made of cheese and Mars isn't just a candy bar.

And computers? The Internet? So common today that young children challenge their elders. Even weirder, with all this going on, while man has almost stripped the Tree of Knowledge bare, he still does not fully understand the workings of the human mind. We've using the mind we *don't understand* to prove things we've *theorised*; things we want to understand. So ask yourself. From where does this mental power come? Have we invented powerful computers without knowing how they work? No! That would be impossible but it has happened! Man has succeeded without fully understanding his own brain. He's put the cart before the horse or, maybe, the space capsule *behind* the rocket?

Our inquiring mind has sidestepped the problem of knowing how we think to prove what we think, that which we've theoriszed. We've done that and we've succeeded but I suspect we've gone about it the wrong way. Maybe *there* lies our mistake. Maybe that's the caveat. What if we're not meant to know? Like the Tower of Babel? Why did the descendents of Noah need to build a tower if not to reach to heaven and to converse with G-d? To understand

Him?   It didn't work. All they did was stop people from communicating freely with each other. Suddenly, they couldn't understand each other.   They began to babble (Babel?). Truth or fable? Fact or fiction? You decide.

But aren't we doing the same? Aren't we building other towers? We might speak different languages but we understand each other's mathematics. So what's to stop these new towers? The Internet? Satellites? Not language; we've "progressed" beyond that. Maybe greed or ambition? The frenzy for power? A fierce desire that'll lead the way to Armageddon; the final battle between good and evil prophesied to end the world. Armageddon. From the Hebraic words, 'har' for mountain and 'Megiddo', the mountain region of Megiddo.   It was a tall mountain – perhaps the tower to oblivion? Food for thought?

Now you're asking yourself what this declamation has to do with depression? My answer? Everything and then some. This is what it's all about. I'm showing you how your mind can operate. Because while you're thinking you're also working on your depression. And it's interesting. So don't leave it all to the scientists. As it is, they're not getting us very far in the survival stakes. Not when it comes to nuclear and   environmental threats.   To global warming things surpassed only by mans' greed. So think and theorise. Form opinions on anything you choose. Oil? HIV/Aids? The financial crisis; another mans' special. invention. Consider whatever you've got a gripe about. You don't want to publish your thoughts and you're not looking for a publisher so think away. You've got a mind so use it. Give it the work out it so badly needs.

After that long detour, it's back to your routine regimen. Not into bed. After exiting that womb, I'd have a bath and plan my day while in the tub; my other womb. It's important to plan because you're confused when you're depressed. You desperately need order in your life because confusion, in an uncertain mindset, can be chaotic. In the tub I'd decide what to wear that day so that, when I was out and drying, I didn't have to suffer the chaos of decision making. Which often becomes instant dilemma, a task too big to handle. In other words, always be one step ahead especially with those trivial things. Avoid confusion and indecision by working out the little things in advance otherwise they'll really mess up your day.

Mornings also mean breakfast and here the same applies. You should already have decided what you're going to eat. If there's someone to prepare breakfast for you, great. We all need support. So discuss it with your partner. I wasn't that lucky but breakfast gave me more opportunity to occupy my mind.

Again, the trick. Use your "spare" time to decide on things then, once that's done, let the day's momentum take over. A phone call or two helps tremendously. No matter how you've dreaded making or taking those calls. Once you've handled them, and handle them you will, stay occupied. Always remember that, excluding certain suicidal connotations, depression is not a life threatening disease although there will be times when you wish it were!

While it's true you can't snap out of your depression, you can use these simple aids to help see you through.

SYMPTOM #2

DETERIORATING QUALITY OF LIFE

Depression really tests your quality of life. You keep asking yourself "what's the point?" When you enjoy sleeping more than doing isn't that another kind of death? It's a tough call when you're in that frame of mind so don't allow those thoughts to manage you. Get occupied! Be with people. Let there be activity about you. That way you'll manage your thoughts more easily.

Let's think about "quality of life" for a moment. It's about your attitude to certain senses or situations. Each one different but no less important. You may not agree with what follows but it's my two cents worth so you're going to get it.

But please, question whatever I say because it is good to question, good to think things out for yourself.

I believe quality of life hinges on certain basics: eating, sleeping, sex, creativity, recreation and job satisfaction. You may not agree with the sex part but I'm sure Sigmund Freud would have been there with me.

Eating. Anxiety and depression bring about changes in your feeding pattern. It will either put you off food entirely or you'll binge. Beware. Because eating disorders can affect you. You won't feel good if you're bloated or if your stomach thinks your throat has been cut.   And you don't have to go on any kind of diet either. Which reminds me of the story of the overweight guy who went on a wine diet. In the first week he lost three days!

Feeling good is what life should be about so if you've got problems with your teeth or dentures, it can only add to the problem.   Like animals, mans' natural inclination is to forage. Is there a greater pleasure than tucking into a favourite meal while hoping it will never end. Like a bottomless cup of coffee. What is life without the joys of food? Never mind about eating to live or living to eat; it doesn't have to be gluttony. Just real pleasure. So what do you do when an eating disorder affects your quality of life?

If you've lost your appetite, plan your meals. Choose those foods you'd best like to eat, those meals you've always put aside for some special day. In other words, get involved with your food planning. If you're out of ingredients, go to the supermarket yourself and buy what you need. If you're not sure what you need, turn up a few recipes. Or check out the Internet. Or just think it through. That's the way to get involved. Remember, *your* taste buds will benefit from your efforts. Again, the flip side. If you're bingeing, you may suffer from constipation. But more about that elsewhere.

Sleeping. Depression can change your sleep patterns. You're either tossing about to get to sleep or you're already awake and your bedside clock is telling you it's still on the wrong side of midnight even though you feel like you've been sleeping for a week. To make things worse, it's a Catch 22. While you enjoy sleeping, being out for the count stops you anticipating those bed hours still ahead before the dreaded wake up call. Be it radio or TV, bugler or bathroom, the call means the same thing. Anticipation of those remaining hours is what you lose when you're asleep but you can't have it both ways. So why are we humans so ridiculously complex?

Sleep is paramount. You feel wonderful after a good night's rest. It clears your head and tops up your energy. So how do we beat the sleep kinks? It's not a problem when you think about it. Solution: Don't go to bed too early. Stay awake longer; ultimately, everyone must sleep. You're thinking it's easy to say but difficult to do? Maybe so but only because getting into bed has become the high point of your day. Much as you hate getting up in the morning, you reward yourself by getting into bed earlier and earlier. Don't! Stay up longer. Read. Do something constructive. Like planning your tomorrow. You sleep better when you're mentally tired.

Creativity. There's nothing more satisfying than being creative. It works for everyone, with anything. Like painting a wall or a picture. Recording a moment. Writing. Designing. Sculpting. Gardening. Working wood. Building a model. Photography. Whatever your talents allow and wherever it takes you. Maybe sport is your thing? Remember, when you're enjoying yourself you're also eyeballing depression. I've said it before. Mental stuff is gym-work for the mind. You may not be pumping iron. Instead, you're pumping thoughts and Ideas. And you're strategising. You're fighting off those negatives, allowing your mind to re-balance. You're tuning into life again, tuning in to life as you used to know it. You're shoving depression behind you with every mental push. Get thee behind me, Satan!

Recreation also has a lot to do with aspects of life we've already discussed. Above all, recreation (a.k.a leisure) recharges your mental batteries and allows you to cope.

Mental stress is far more taxing than the physical equivalent. Recreation is like being on vacation. You're occupying your mind in different ways. And there's direction in all this because whichever way you use your mind, you're on the cure route. By merely concentrating on things.

While it is your the principle organ, think of your brain as a muscle you exercise just by thinking. Or by reading. There are many excellent mind exercises so choose. None of them are *erg* dependant.

There's nothing better than meditation. I've often wondered about the depression rate of Zen Buddhists. Any folk who meditate. I bet it doesn't even figure.

Chess is another good exercise. Or card games like bridge. Anything that keeps the mind alert will keep depression at a distance. The choice is endless.

<u>Sex.</u> By far the ultimate creative experience. And not necessarily in the variations or positions you might conjure! Sex is the most essential joy. Has so been meant because the act creates life itself. As the Good Book commands, go forth and multiply.

Sadly, anxiety and depression can ravage your libido and what is left if you can't, or don't, enjoy sex? When it's too much trouble to even get aroused? When the very thought of foreplay makes you yawn, want to turn over and go to sleep. It can get to that and when it does, you tell yourself you're not human anymore. What's the point when sex isn't what it used to be and you can't eat, think or sleep properly either? Hell, what happened to whatever turned life into a wonderland? Now that was quality of life!

Don't overdo the guilt bit. Sex is important but it isn't everything. You're not an adult male lion who eats and seeps all day and demands the right to fornicate whenever it suits him. Who is so lazy his lionesses have to hunt for food and he has the audacity to eat his fill first, leaving barely enough for the others in the pride. Even for his cubs. If that's what you mean by quality of life, then you have my sympathy because somewhere you've lost the way. Life is more than a hedonistic journey so use your mind to get above it. Read, study, plan and ponder. As much as you're obsessed with depression, balance your brain. Gather food for the soul. Knowledge has always been the mainstay of life. Again another dichotomy. The more you know the more you realise how little you know. Or how much there is to know.

It's a state of mind. Like the nonagenarian who asked his doctor to lower his sex urge. "Lower it?" asked the incredulous doctor. "You're ninety three!" "Yes," insisted the patient. "Lower it from my mind to my penis."

You should use your mind to face up to and triumph over what is going on in *your* brain. Being clever is a state of mind so fight any cranium imbalance with your intellect. Let your determination lead. Plan. Strategise. Be that one mental stride ahead. In other words, be clever!

SYMPTOM #3
WHERE'S THE LAUGHTER?

Have you heard of anything more frivolous? Laughter? When we're discussing depression? It may be strange but it's true. I used to laugh a lot. Genuine laughter. I enjoyed a good joke, remembered them all and passed them on, laughed more and more the second, third and even the fourth time around. In fact I may have overdone it because my every sentence ended with a chuckle. Maybe I was inventing my own version of Victor Borge's delightful "phonetic punctuation" nonsense. Whatever it was, it did me a world of good because no-one likes a grump. People will shy away from you if, like Atlas, you're forever carrying the world on your shoulders.

Your laugh is you. It sparks your personality, induces a glitter which is your own kind of magnetism and keeps it shining through. The world is supposed to laugh with you so help it along. Very often, even a smile is enough but when you get people laughing, you're rebuilding the confidence depression has taken from you.

What if you've never been a "laugher"? Developing a good, honest laugh sounds like a contradiction. No matter. You'll begin to see the funny, the less serious side of things. Here's an example. I had just been diagnosed with testicular cancer. I remember so well sitting across the urologist's desk. He was a swarthy, very serious sort with thick, bushy black eyebrows and a droopy black moustache that weighed down from his nose. Thinking back, he may also have been depressed. Although my knees were knocking, I understood his situation. Having to tell people they had cancer wasn't a whole lot of fun. While I was certainly not the first one he'd told, it still wasn't going to be the laugh of the century. Then, after he told me, after my initial shock; I was sure his moustache had drooped further, what the hell, I thought. There was nothing I could do about it. *He* was the uro. *He* was supposed to see me through the problem. Wasn't that why I'd gone to see him? Then suddenly the enormity of it hit and all I had left was a laugh. Sure. I know. The thin line between comedy and tragedy but I did laugh and it saw me through.

My first cancer operation was fourteen years ago. My last some months behind me as I write so don't tell me laughter didn't play a role. Sure, it didn't cure my cancer but neither did it harm my morale. So, I urge you, face up to depression with whatever humour you can gather. Give it your best shot because laughter lifts the soul, adds fizz to your personality and boosts your confidence. Look for the funnier things. There's always something you can latch on to. Humour is like music. What would life be without music? Even if you've never laughed, try it out. Start from the beginning. With a smile. There's power in a smile. It'll get you going and the rest will follow. The more often you smile the easier it gets. It's easier to smile than to scowl, easier to be nice than to be nasty. So be nice and smile. Kids will tell you the longest word in the English language is "smiles". Because there's a mile between the 'esses'.

SYMPTOM #4
REDUCED LIBIDO

We're back to this one. Libido is one of those items leading to things "once enjoyed". Depression can do this to you either because of depression itself or because it's a side effects of the medication you're on. Maybe it's not too worrisome for you. It depends on the person you are. To me it was more than a mental thing because of my testicular cancer problem. My wife having died a few years before, I was on my own after many years and into my sixth year of loneliness. Every time I closed the front door, I'd shut the world out behind me. So, I finally decided. Enough! Being a lonesome widower was for losers. Sure, as much as I yearned for her, I couldn't get my wife back so I found a lady friend. Or she found me; I'm not quite sure. Someone I had dated in my teens. Chunkier now. But I wasn't the Adonis I'd never been. So who cared?

She had a delightful sense of humour – laughed at all my jokes - but had an insatiable need to be out. Movies, dinners, opera, orchestra. Jazz bands. Lectures. Anything and everything motivated her. Which really wasn't my scene but it certainly got me out of my rut.

Of all the things I tried, being with people helped the most. It was great getting phone calls and hearing someone ask how I was doing. Had I had taken my tablets? How was I going to spend my day?. I'd fetch her or she'd come over. so I started cooking again. I'd open a bottle of wine and we'd have a glass or two. I'd prepare oven baked fish with white wine and butter sauce. Or pasta alla principessa (my own melange of Italian recipes I particularly enjoy). Sometimes filleted chicken with fried banana and a pinch of curry on a creamy bed of rice. And of course, my very own onion soup. Better than the Parisian, even if I say so myself which was strange because I found the recipe in an Italian cook book! Is Paris in Italy?

Once, when in Vienna, I specially ordered wiener schnitzel because it was Vienna and I had to taste the real thing. I still believe my schnitzel is better so I call it schnitzel a la Cap. Yes, I prepared dishes like that. Nothing ever approaching haute cuisine. More like *cuisine bourgeois* I thought - even that may be giving me more than my due - but it tasted good and it was fun. We'd either go to the movies then eat out or stay indoors and enjoy my 'palate-stimulating' delights. Maybe watch the occasional good movie on television then go downstairs to the foyer restaurant for decaff and chocolate or cheese cake. Yes. It was good to be alive again.

SYMPTOM #5

THOUGHTS OF SUICIDE
[a k a WHAT'S THE POINT TO IT ALL?]

This is serious stuff. In this frame of mind you're not thinking 'where there's life there's hope' but 'where there's hope there's life'. Or what's the point?   Quite common when everything seems too much. How well I know those feelings of hopelessness. What's the point when all you want is to do is opt out? When suicide seems the 'logical' way out and the more you think about it, the more appealing it gets. You ask yourself, "Is it the answer?" Then you think about how you'd do it. A pill overdose; a more gentle end but it takes time and time is courage. Especially then. A bullet, maybe? Quick but so messy. What about jumping off a building? No. You're afraid of heights! Drowning? Ghastly. Carbon monoxide poisoning?   Maybe.   Or driving off a cliff? Strangely in that state of mental turbulence, dying isn't so bad at all which, I suppose, is depression's macabre way of preparing you for when your time does eventually run out.

So it gets you thinking that perhaps depression is a cure in itself, like the common cold was once suspected to be. Which must mean that death can't be all that its cracked up to be! You didn't want to be born so now you want to die.

Sounds reasonable. Maybe death is just the way to that great airport in the sky. Your flight has been booked but the destination is still open. What if there isn't an after life? So you start thinking of it as a big sleep. The big brother sleep to the little sleeps you've been enjoying lately. Except that you only enjoy the sleep once you're awake and you're telling yourself how great it was!

Which reminds me of a TV interview I once saw. The interviewee was that great pianist, Arthur Rubinstein. He was in his nineties at the time and the interviewer asked him. "Do you believe in a life hereafter?" The pianist shook his head. "No," he replied sadly. "And what will you think, if, when you get there you find there *is* a life hereafter?" asked the interviewer. Rubinstein's watery eyes twinkled happily. "I think I shall be delighted," he replied.

When sleep becomes depression's cherry; the thing you best like to do, you'll try to persuade yourself that sleep is a kind of death in itself. Wrong! Know this. Suicide is no way out. You've got to be very mixed up or very brave to take your own life. No-one in their right mind can ever think of surrendering the greatest gift of all? Your problems aside, surely you enjoy the air that you breathe, the sights that you see, the sensations you feel? Especially when tomorrow can be so different? You wouldn't turn down a lottery win so why think of opting out of life when it's greatest gift of all?

Understand that you're depressed and think tomorrow's thoughts. Because every sunrise replicates creation and brings with it a new dawn that should be full of hope. And after a few more tomorrows, all will be well again.

Regretfully, in this mind set attempts at suicide are common. But thinking about it and doing it are often miles apart. Fortunately so. Yet, sadly, suicides do occur even though there's a way out. With all this going on in your mind, especially during those dreadful hours, go back to basics. Think and plan. Let your daily routine see you through. But you *must tell someone* about your mental, your suicidal thoughts. Admit it openly and look for company. Be with people, preferably those you can lean on and confide in. You need the comfort of understanding, compassionate people who will listen to you. Even better, find help. Contact help organisations like Lifeline or whatever its equivalent in your area because they know how to help, are equipped to handle your situation. Knowing you're potentially suicidal, you should have already noted their contact telephone numbers. Suicide isn't just like surviving getting out of bed in the morning. Suicide is forever. It is serious business and you must go to whatever lengths necessary to preserve yourself.

Log on to the Internet. Surf the web. You'll find a lot of help out there so take advantage of it. Do it fast! Don't hesitant because your life is in the balance and you need all the help you can get.

When you're over the hurdle, once you're thinking positively again, everything will be a lot brighter. Again you'll be dealing with your daily matters again which, in itself, is also a cure. But all the while, it's essential to be on medication, essential that you take the prescribed dosage religiously. Talk to your clinician regularly. Your medication may have to be increased. Know that the clinicians can only help if you keep them informed. Finally and above all, know that suicide is contrary to everything we believe and it is not for you. Because, I repeat, suicide is forever.

SYMPTOM #6
NEED FOR MEDICATION OR THERAPY:

We already know that depression isn't something you can snap out of on your own, that you need the support of your loved ones; the warmth of family and friends; people. Even with this people support, know that the most important support system is effective medication. Whatever suits your metabolism. I was on Prozac – fluoxetine - which seems to have more generic derivatives than any other. It seems that fluoxetine is most effective. The normal dosage is 20 mg daily. However, it takes a few weeks for the drug to start it's magic but when it's on, it helps enormously. While not a panacea, it certainly allows you to add your own input, your personality, hopefully your *joie de vivre,* to the healing process. My house doctor started me on 20 mg Prozac daily. It kicked in after a few weeks but not as well as I thought so he referred me to a psychiatrist who immediately upped the dose to 30 mg which evened out the kinks. Since then, I've been up to 40 mg but eventually leveled out at a daily 20 mg.

It doesn't have to be Prozac. Not even fluoxetine. There are many other good anti-depressants around. You've just got to find the one that suits you best at, hopefully, the right price. The professionals know because that's their job. Sure there are also other procedures and psychotherapies. Often in combination. So speak to the practitioners. They know all about SSRIs [selective serotonin reuptake inhibitors] about MAOIs [monoamine oxidase inhibitors] and TCAs [tricyclic anti-depressants]. And don't forget the SNRIs [serotonin-norepinephrine re-uptake inhibitors]. All of which I know less than nothing about so I won't bore you with that kind of talk. Just know that your medical people do know and, if they don't, they'll refer you to someone who does. There are many shrinks and psychologists. Their field of expertise is mental health matters. Not only serious mental problems. They have a lot to do with depression. There being so many of us victims, depression to them is what seasonal flu is to the GP. You could say, depression is the shrink's bread and butter. Hopefully not Shakespeare's "caviary to the general."

As I understand it, unlike a psychologist, a psychiatrist is a medical specialist who can prescribe anti-depressants and all other drugs. So he's the pro who will determine the most effective regimen for you, something that works best with the least side effects. At first the shrink's approach may seem like guesswork but that is not so. He has to start you on what he thinks is the best drug for you. But it may not be effective so he'll try something else. It may take a while but once he has found a drug that suits, he will establish your dosage. And instruct you not to stop taking it or change anything without consultation. Also, in the beginning, you may think the stuff's not working when, in reality, it hasn't even kicked in yet. And later, when you're feeling a lot better, you may think you don't need it anymore. Don't ever do anything rash and always be in touch with your practitioners and let them know how you are doing. Know also that you may have to stay on anti-depressants for quite a while. Never do anything that may jolt you back to square one.

The message is clear. Never stop your anti-depressant medication or change the dosage without first speaking to your practitioners. Also, if they want you to go off the medication, they will explain how you may safely do so.

Those of us with bi-polar or major chronic depression may have to stay on medication indefinitely. Above all, think of your medication as the very foundation of your cure.

I'm not *au fait* with homeopathic or naturopathic remedies although I have heard that Selenium, a non-metallic element, discovered by the Swedish chemist Baron Jons Jakob Bezelius (he also discovered Thorium and Cerium and coined the word "protein") has been found to be effective. However, if you prefer the "natural" route, ask your consultant for advice before you do anything.   Whatever remedy you choose, *if it works,* believe in it.

SYMPTOM #7
CONFUSION: DECISION MAKING CONCENTRATING, MEMORY LAPSES.

These symptoms are nothing more than negative mental calisthenics but what do you expect? You're depressed because you have a mind problem. If you're suffering these symptoms without being depressed you may have a problem, could be suffering from something like Alzheimer's, which, relative to your age, could be an associated illness sometimes hidden by depression. But that's not for me to judge or advise. Just know that all symptom #7 items are "par for the course" for depression.

We've already discussed the problems we have with small decisions. So, if you are dithering over the small fry, you'll be thrown when you start grappling with the more important ones which are usually lurking nearby. Understand, you can't opt out of everything because you're depressed. Nor can you, as some folk say, go through life enjoying yourself. Which is probably why depression was invented.   Along with dentists, lawyers and architects! Which suggests a story I heard the other day. About this guy who walked into a bar and shouted, "All lawyers are assholes!" Silence. Then, from the back, a voice.   "I take exception to that remark." "Why," asked the first guy. "You a lawyer?" "No," came the reply. "I'm an asshole!"

So stay with me. Humour won't hurt.

Back to the present. So what do you do about this decision making thing? Here's what. Have a cup of something to help you relax while you're carefully thinking about the problem. That done, jot the problem down. Then draw a vertical line down the centre of the page. Head the one column "PROS" and the other column "CONS". The PROS are your reactions that have positive advantages, the CONS those with negative connotations. Take your time.

Think of the various aspects of the problem, write them down and keep pondering. Examine all the possible answers and note them down in the appropriate column. Then, when you're done, give a single point to each answer and add each column. Obviously the highest score will win. But that's not it. Once you know the score, let your gut have the final say. I know you're thinking it's a tortuous process but the benefit of this strange method is that it makes you think the matter through very, very thoroughly. Another advantage is that you were thinking logically, your thoughts were ordered and attuned and then you allowed the inner-you to make the final decision.

Remembering, of course, that *there is no perfect decision.* To everything there's an advantage and a disadvantage which, I suppose, could be another Newtonian Law.

Remember. Always try to be one step ahead of the race. Tackle your difficulty *before* it becomes a problem. They're part of life so they'll always be around but try to anticipate them before the mound becomes a mountain. Think ahead and try to avoid difficulties, don't invite them to tea.

Very often, problems solve themselves while you're working through the processes. Like what happened to me when, very depressed, I was running a major building project with a hot contractor on my tail and an impossible client running the sidelines while I couldn't hold a pen in my hand. Yet had to remember stacks of technical details. Somehow, I managed. Having to take instant decisions at well attended site meetings with professionals and contractors present in numbers with everyone eager to pounce is never a joy even when you're not depressed. But you manage because depression has *only shrouded* you ability. Depression can never *deprive* you of your abilities.

Which indicates that decision making is linked to your confidence level that, in the good old pre-depression days, always saw you through. Your confidence may now be more fuzzy but it's still there and the power of your brain cells is unaffected. You've always known and relied on your ability. You know what you have achieved in the past and will again achieve. So while depression may try to whittle away your confidence and may even reduce you to a relic of yourself *in a stressed situation,* it cannot pirate your ability! Therefor, prepare yourself for what's ahead the best way you can. Get clever! Try to anticipate the problems, snags and questions that might be thrown at you. Even if yours is only a half hearted attempt, a gesture, it'll help you think things through.

"But how is that possible?" you cry. "I'm depressed. I can't think!" You can think. And in a tight situation you will think. Your mind will rise above depression and provide the answers. You'll rise above your depression and extricate yourself from the mess because in facing the problem head on, your mind has forced depression into a back seat. And it proves that your ability, your desire to succeed, has not been undermined. Under pressure, you'll do great things and like the Phoenix, that *rara avis*, you will rise from the ashes. Sadly, only to find yourself back on the pyre the next day. But that's how it goes.

The whole spiel is a matter of constant mind work, sometimes difficult but worth it in the end. And necessary because it has to be done. And every time you succeed, as you will, that's another rung up the confidence ladder, another step up to normality. You're already feeling better in yourself. You're feeling better and facing the future with greater determination

Now let's talk about concentrating. What? You say you can't concentrate? Surprise! Surprise! Of course you can't. Because you haven't been concentrating on anything but mundane TV shows for how long? And that's hardly concentrating. Dear reader, dear fellow victim, to concentrate effectively you've got to *retrain your mind*. I went back to university when I was a mature student of 34 summers, hadn't held a text book, hadn't taken a note since my last year in high school when I was sixteen. And because I hadn't concentrated on anything academic for eighteen years, I did something about it.

"Varsity?" you say. That's not the concentration you had in mind. OK. I agree. But the principle is the same. It is pointless going to the gym to just go through the motions. Hell, you'll do more good staying home to mow the lawn. Or do the dishes.

So how do you learn to concentrate? You don't *learn* to concentrate. You put yourself in situations where you have got to understand things and where understanding only comes through concentration. Concentration is not like re-learning to ride a bike. It's very different. Your mind must be sharpened because it has become sluggish through lack of use. It must be nurtured. So get some books from your local library, something more than easy reading. Choose topics you've always wanted to know more about. Then read and learn. It'll stimulate your mind. Get into reading then move on, try something more difficult, more challenging but stay away from subjects too complicated. Unless they're your bent. To help me concentrate again, I decided to go through the entire math syllabus I had done in school. I bought the latest text and answer books, put my rear end on a chair and got down to it because I had been told a good knowledge of mathematics was a prerequisite for my studies. I mean, I had math but it was rusty. So I did it all again.

In a different vein, I knew very little about philosophy and wanted to know more. So I got hold of phil books and read. Now I know a little more about Descartes and his *"cogito ergo sum"*. And a little more about some of the other great thinkers. Not much but more than I knew before. Enough to keep me concentrating and to keep me enthralled. I never tried Einstein's *"E = MC etc"* because, understandably, he was way above me. His was a great intellect. Sadly not mine but it led me to astronomy and the wonders of the universe. Fascinating stuff.

In relearning how to concentrate, I was reminded of something important. We all know that the more you put into something, the more you'll get out of it. Forget the "no pain no gain" thing. There was no pain in learning. Just a lot of gain.

So get thinking. I spoke to a lovely person the other day. She was once a depressive. We were talking about concentrating and she explained how, in her worst moments, she would take up to take up to thirty minutes to peel a single potato! An half hour of sheer concentration for that simple task. She wasn't on medication, she admitted, which, I suppose, explains some of it. But it was a complete mind game to her. Something she willed herself to do and achieve it she did. That's all long behind her now. She's still lovely and delightful to be with; the epitome of a natural person. Full of fun and laughter. You'd never say she was once a victim.

Now for memory lapses. This happens to all of us. if you're a senior, you'll know it as a "senior moment." Which isn't fair because I don't recall meaningful "junior moments". With me it was names to begin with. I mean, after spending "on the job" years with people, came the day that I suddenly couldn't remember their names. Impossible? No, it happens! OK, so it comes back later but not when you need it most. Like the time I landed up at an ambassadorial cocktail party and was chatting to a senator when a socially inclined person joined us. I knew she wanted to meet the senator which wasn't possible because I'd forgotten his name! I was cornered and in a cold sweat and had to start the introduction. The lady first (thank goodness I remembered who she was) then it was the senator's turn. I suddenly saw a way out. When just about to name the senator, I broke into a fit of coughing! So he finished it for me, introduced himself and all was well. It was close and, again, it highlights the adage, "If you can't be strong, be clever!" Even though there was canniness in what I did!

You may forget the date Kennedy was assassinated. But can you forget that President's name? Yes, you can and there's a good chance you will. As one gets older, the grey cells seem less responsive. Could be Alzheimer's or Parkinson's. The latter is brought on because the dopamine producing brain cells die off. Parkinson's, the encylopaedia also tells me, can be associated with depression but then so many other things are as well so there's no cause for alarm. By all means, get it checked out if you feel you must.

If you can't remember, make notes. Don't rely on memory because every thought introduces others which keep twirling in your brain like noisy buttons in a clothes drier. If you list your problems, you'll find the inventory a lot less daunting than you imagined and easier to handle. If you can't remember names, use keywords; associate words. Then you only have to worry about remembering the keywords! But jokes aside, recently, I had trouble remembering the word "travertine". So I associated it with "Trevor", an erstwhile friend. Trevor = travetine. Close enough. Get it? Use any keywords that come to mind. What you choose isn't important. What is important is that you keep your mind active because, if you don't, depression will slow it down further.

Above all, don't spend your hours watching TV. Read instead. When you're into a story, you're creating images, converting the written word into mind pictures without sharply defined outlines. That's why we're usually disappointed when we see the movie of a book we've enjoyed. Because someone has brazenly replaced our slant to the author's imagination with scenes quite different. Reading is far more enjoyable than watching a screen. Or being engrossed in those half hours of myth and mayhem, of death destruction and devilry known as 'The News'. Also I prefer not to listen to filthy language. To me, that ain't 'entertainment'.

Your imagination is a powerful tool. Use it wisely because it's therapeutic and that's just what you need right now. Einstein is supposed to have said something about the average human only needing a spine because he hardly used his brain. So don't waste your mind. Relegate the television to the back room – maybe even the garage - because, in my opinion, that is where it should stay. Sure, I'm knocking TV. For reasons of sanity.

Want my advice? When you're depressed, limit your time in front of the box. Rediscover your mental assets by using your brain and discarding TV's detritus.

SYMPTOM #8

SEVERE TENSION AND STRESS

I'd be surprised if you did NOT suffer from tension and stress. These things gang up on you even when you're "normal" so why should they disappear when you're depressed? Like inflation, depression is one big run around. Its gloom contaminates your very existence leading to heightening tension and stress even if you are on tranquilisers. Because those are only effective for about four hours although there are others long action types which do the trick if you disregard the weird things that can happen to you.

While tranquilisers can limit stress, a major player in the depression cycle, they don't do much for depression. I quote Mary Wollstonecraft Shelley who, circa 1850, said, "Nothing contributes so much to tranquilise the mind as a steady purpose." In other words, be occupied.

However, my shrink did prescribe a long action, 24 hour, non-addictive tranquiliser. He smiled and casually remarked, "Be careful with it. Strange things may happen." I was too far gone to argue so I took the medication for the short period prescribed and it worked very well. In fact, it cured all those unexplained physical disorders that had obviously been induced by stress. Incidently, I have a theory about the consequences of stress. I believe very strongly that stress is the root cause of all our physical, social and emotional problems.

Regarding the physical, I believe that any part of the body subjected to constant stress is under threat because it is sufficiently weakened to invite disease. In my case, it was cancer. Take my lymphoma of the sartorius muscle. It was constantly under stress. When I was driving, my left foot was always hovering above the clutch pedal; yes, I'm an old fashioned guy. Also when getting in and out of my Mini car and at home, getting in and out of a deep narrow bath without handles. Instead of a handle, I became a contortionist, used my left leg to lever myself in and out of the bath. That's why I thought the swelling on the inside of my thigh was just a strain. Later it was identified as a lymphoma. This isn't a medical theory or one that would be remotely supported by the medical fraternity but I'm convinced I'm right. Why, I ask, did lymphoma attack my sartorius muscle; the last place anyone would suspect. Unless, in terms of my theory, *that* muscle was vulnerable.

SYMPTOM #9
PESSIMISM & FEELINGS OF HOPELESSNESS

Because it hinders achievement, this is another natural reaction to depression Something is stopping you from coming out on top, from accomplishing those things you've been doing all your life. What do you do about it? Firstly, think of this as another aspect of trauma. Again, not life threatening but very distressing because sudden change in lifestyle can be traumatic.

When these symptoms manifest, remind yourself that you've always accomplished whatever you set out to do. Now something is holding you back. What is making life difficult? Why can everyone else be cheerful except you? Others can smile, can be useful, can work, can serve a purpose. Everyone but you! Understand this is just another piece of depression's jigsaw. So tell yourself it will come right when you regain normality. Above all, don't stress about it. It'll go when your depression ends.

SYMPTOM #10
DISINTEREST IN ACTIVITIES ONCE ENJOYED

What a perplexing monster this is. You have already asked why you suddenly turned away from those things you used to reish? Which, in my case, was spending time on the beach, year in and year out, summer through winter, reveling in the invigorating Atlantic chill. In the company of friends crazy enough to enjoy the same. The beach was across the road from my apartment so getting there wasn't a problem yet depression was strong enough to keep me away. And keep me away it did for a long time. I became couch bound and watched Oprah. Never missed a session with Dr. Phil and followed up with the soaps! What had happened to me?

How did I solve the problem? I got involved with people again. It didn't come easy. In the beginning, I had to work at it but it was worth it. There's no better therapy than being with friends, swopping yarns. Laughing, talking, listening. Just being.

When you're depressed, being alone is the worst. Loneliness is bad news. Having too much time on your hands is a bad mistake because it broods negative thoughts that'll rack you from dusk to dawn. So, accept an invitation for a chat. Or for drinks, cards, whatever. Then invite people over and enjoy their company because if you're alone, doom clouds will engulf you.

SYMPTOM #11
BAD "NERVES", TREMOURS, JUMPINESS

This was a menace. I'd jump at every noise. Even the telephone was a major hazard. I was out of my skin whenever it rang. Not only because of the noise. It meant I had to answer.

Depression gave me tremours and I shook. Drinking my morning tea was a messy two-handed effort. Also, the shakes kept me away from people because I was embarrassed about it. I dreaded eating or drinking in public. Friends or strangers, it made no difference. And it was the same when I had to write. Even signing my credit card voucher in the supermarket was a mission. Isn't that ridiculous?

But I know, now, that I was also suffering from "social phobia disorder". (Read more about it in Section II under "Symptoms of Anxiety Disorders.") Seems I was getting depression's full treatment with no holds barred. Just think about it for a moment! Why was I embarrassed? What difference did it make to anyone? Who cares if you shake? Who would possibly be interested and if they were, so what!? I was shaking, wasn't infecting anyone so shake, baby, shake.

What did I do about it? I had it checked out and, thankfully, it wasn't a problem so I opted for admission. Whenever I was with someone, I'd deliberately draw attention to my shaking. Like the Alcoholics Anonymous introduction. "My name is John Smith and I'm an alcoholic." I even told the old joke about the guy in the bar who shook so badly he spilt most of his drinks. Noticing, the barman remarked. "You drink a lot?" "No," came the reply, "I spill a lot!"

I found that the only way to overcome these problems was to get out and do it. So I told my lady friend all about it.

Understandably, her first reaction was to laugh. Because it was that ridiculous but then she helped me through it. She would suggest restaurants where we could find a darker corner, even suggested I drink coffee or wine through a straw!

That was then. I got over it a long time ago. How? I suppose it decided it'd had had enough of me. It was one of those things that came and went with depression. Now I go everywhere. I eat and drink and enjoy myself as I haven't done for years. When depressed, I'd have a glass of wine. Or two; I discussed it with my GP - because alcohol and anti-depressants don't go well together - and he gave me the nod. "In moderation," he said. I know alcohol didn't stop me shaking but the shakes didn't affect me any more which was great.

Having the shakes doesn't only affect your eating and drinking. It also affects holding things, like pens and pencils or working the computer. Stopping the cursor jump was a challenge. I had always been meticulous when it came to my handwriting. It had to look and be good, had been like that ever since I learned how so when I started to shake, everything changed and I was shattered. I couldn't sign my name in front of people so I developed an untidy squiggle that was easy to do. Now, fortunately, those ridiculous moments are over and I sign my name with aplomb. Like before. Because I am me. I am who I am. What had Descartes said? *Cogito ergo sum.* I think therefore I am. Why not me too? I can think and I can write and my signature proves it.

SYMPTOM #12
UNEXPLAINED PHYSICAL DISORDERS

Depression is comfortable with stress and stress begets skin disorders. Nasty ones, like psoriasis. I know because both hit me at the same time. I used to pride myself on my skin. I was without blemish *then suddenly I was one big blemish.* Psoriasis raided my body. Chest, back and legs. Especially on my shins, scalp and elbows. Thinking back, it's possible my skin disorder was one of the reasons I stayed away from the beach which was the wrong thing to do because ultra violet light is supposed to do great things for psoriasis though some might disagree. Isn't it strange that most times, depression is easier to cure than psoriasis!

I consulted dermatologists and tried their medications but nothing worked and because tar-based concoctions were so messy, I steered clear of them. Unexpectedly, chemotherapy did the magic. Methotrexate in the chemotherapy cocktail is used to treat psoriasis. As a precaution, you must have your liver and kidney functions checked regularly before ingestion but as that's standard practice when you're on chemo, I took the medication and it worked.   Some of the marks remained but the lesions disappeared. Which means chemotherapy is a perk. As my oncologist remarked. "We may take your hair but we will fix your psoriasis."

I was also having trouble with my back and stomach. Whenever I stood for longer than a few moments, a steel band would clamp my stomach and lower back forcing me to sit. Another 'unexplained' physical disorder was constipation. At first the doctor thought it might be a medication side effect so off I went to a specialist who checked and shunted me to the radiologist for a barium enema. I suppose I shouldn't judge but the last thing I needed at that time was a gut full of barium's gummy, viscous, constipating goo. But I suffered the procedure and was pronounced clean. I mention these problems here because they responded to the long acting tranquiliser the shrink prescribed. Within forty eight hours, the constipation had solved itself and my lower back and stomach muscles had relaxed. I could stand again. I could move around with ease. I was still depressed but without those unexplained aches and pains.

The long-action tranquiliser was weird. Going to the bathroom one night, I found myself on my back on the floor. It was mid-summer and the tiles were cool against my skin so I lay there for a few moments before I realised that I shouldn't be there. Not prone on the floor. I still don't know how it had happened or how I'd fallen but fallen I had because there was no other way I could have ended up there.   Thinking about it, I shuddered.   I could have smashed my skull against the bath. Or the wash basins. I could have done myself a serious injury.

What had happened? It could only have been the tranquilisers and those so called "strange" things the shrink had so casually warned me about. But if you ask me which I preferred? Unexplained physical disorders like constipation and lower back strain, I'll take the tranquiliser every time because they certainly worked.

Then, again, some of us suffer from diarrhea; the other end of the scale. Which is better? Or worse? I don't know and it's not a topic I enjoy discussing but I've learned that if you're going to have treatment, like chemotherapy, or anything that may cause constipation, be proactive. Take a slow acting laxative in advance and prevent a huge problem. However, if your constipation is already chronic, don't go the slow route. Get a laxative that works quickly. But always speak to your doctor.

I talk about my experiences throughout this little book to explain what I've gone through. I'm implying that you could suffer the same so please don't think of this as a personal history. Regard it rather as things that can happen to you, incidents that stayed with me and formulated the tips and suggestions contained in these pages.

SYMPTOM #13
FATIGUE & LETHARGY
[a.k.a. LACK OF MOTIVATION OR INITIATIVE]

You can trace this one back to early morning "get-out-of-bed" syndrome and to changed sleep patterns. As previously explained, some of the symptoms can be 'lumped' together when we consider management strategy. Again we return to the secret: being mentally occupied and staying like that. I know that fatigue and lethargy won't help engross you in anything. However, they remain part of depression's distressing symptoms, may be slow moving adjuncts but prepare your mind to accept them and decide how to overcome them while you're planning. Again, it's the mind game so give it all you've got. Understand that you've only got to *make a move* towards the problem. Once you've overcome inertia, nature will take it's course. Things will happen and you'll be away.

There is another way to get motivated. Set yourself goals. We all want something and it matters not what it is as long as you want it enough and don't covet. I wanted a new car because I was done with what I had and depression, because of medical bills, had used up the cash I'd put away for it.   In my case it was a car.   Maybe you want to get married or feel you need a vacation. Set your goal and plan but first study the situation from all angles and then act. Sure, there'll be stops along the way but it can be done if you're hungry enough and realistic. Be systematic in your planning. Set the challenges and reward yourself when you get to each base. Even if it's only a kind word to yourself, a mental pack on the back. It's important to acknowledge that your plans are working out. Depressions' beast will always crumble against confrontation.

Depression only flourishes where inactivity and negativity prevail but it can't match determined, opposition. Depression *wants* you to stay in bed, wants you to be miserable and without motivation. Think of Newton's Third Law of Motion about their being a reaction to each and every action. If lying in bed is the action, the obvious reaction is to get out of there. So throw aside the covers and get going.

During my study years, to get out of bed I'd throw my legs in the air and yell "I won't graduate by lying on my butt!" And I wasn't even depressed then. Which means I needed those words so much more when I was depressed. Get this into your noggin. You won't beat depression lying on your butt!

SYMPTOM #14
PERSONAL   HYGIENE   &   GENERAL APPEARANCE

This is perhaps the easiest trap of all. It seems such a schlep to wash or bath or shower. Just the thought of brushing your teeth is enough to make you want to abdicate the world and afterwards, you've still got to decide what to wear. And what to eat. Yes, I know. You don't want any part of it!

But by now you're beginning to sense the logic in these pages because here it is again.   The morning syndrome.   The mind game that we've discussed *ad nauseum*.   But because it's important, let me remind you again. You should have already planned and arranged your day so your mind is already confronting your problems. Suddenly you realise you're standing up to more than one symptom. You're holding your own against more than one problem and you're winning!

It'll helps to be presentable.   Because there is something special about feeling good in your clothes, being cool or hip or neat. Whatever. When like that, your personal esteem is up. Being well turned out will give you confidence and that's what you need when you're depressed. You can never have enough confidence because it keeps you in front.

So make the most of yourself and know that there's a special quality about achieving. When you're depressed because you're succeeding against odds loaded against you. Look good in the mirror and you'll look better in your mind. It'll show in your achievements.

SYMPTOM #15
LOSS OF SELF ESTEEM:

Loss of initiative, motivation, confidence and self esteem is perhaps the worst trick depression can play on you. It effects your life, makes you sensitive to feelings of uselessness. Of being incapable, being guilty of laziness. You consider yourself a worthless fraud. The tiniest task is a mountain to be moved. Like CFS, chronic fatigue syndrome, this feeling is very real. Not true but real! So what do you do about it? I give you a three word answer. *Just do it!*

Whatever it is, do it! Steel yourself, prepare yourself for the mind game because you're the only one who can play it. Prepare yourself mentally a few days ahead. Psyche yourself and get stuck in. It's time to prove yourself! You'll find it will take less effort than you expected. You will find you'll do it with ease. Because you've done it so often before depression got its claws into you. And you always did it well.

This is all part of the recuperative process. The same way fluoxetine gathers in your system before it gets to work, so too do these acts of "duty" gather then build up in your esteem. They prepare you for life after depression so always know, always be aware, that while you're absorbed in your tasks, depression has had to take a back seat. And when you've done whatever you had to do, your spirit will soar.

Loss of self esteem affects everything you do. You look in the mirror and you don't like what you see. You can't decide on anything because you can't think clearly. You're unsure about everything which is ridiculous. How can you be unsure of things you've done a million times before without thinking? Does it make sense? Suddenly you're not sure of things which, before you got depressed, you'd decide on at a mind boggling rate. Without ever doubting yourself. Can it be that you're someone else? A different person? You're hesitant, unsure, confused. A lot of nonsense, of course, but you must face those moments. Look into that mirror and picture what you once were. Because that's who you still are! Convince yourself that you're going to reclaim your image. Feel that you're getting to grips with your depression, that you won't let it control you again. That it's *your* mind and *you* are in control. Recall the things you've done and above all, get moving! Depression cannot survive activity. So get to it and revel in the thrill because now you're doing to depression what it has done to you. And you're winning!

Everything's a mission when you're depressed. You have to work to pay the rent but you can't get going and because you're beaten, you procrastinate. I'm self employed which is not good for depressives because job attendance is more lenient. When you're on a payroll, you've got to be at work on time and you've got to perform; a blessing that keeps you busy and those negative thoughts at bay. So persevere. Sir Winston Churchill said, way back, in 1914, at the beginning of World War I, "Sure I am of this, that you have only to endure to conquer. You have only to persevere to save yourselves."

To get motivated, *plan*. Convince yourself a few days ahead that you're going to do whatever it is you've got to do. That way, when the time comes, you're already committed. You're motivated. You may still think it's a huge task and it may take some doing but you're ready for it. Which is not as bad as having to face something that comes at you out of the blue. So try to anticipate. Try to keep incidents at arms lengths before they turn into problems.

Loss of motivation is a difficult one because you've got to work at it all the time. I guess it's putting one foot in front of the other until you're walking. Motivation is an attitude in itself.   Some folk work better under pressure. They won't suffer anything because they know they'll do it when they must! Which is exactly what everyone out there is doing right now.   They're just getting on with their lives. They may not be depressed but they're also only coping because they're not magicians. Not heroes. They're getting by albeit without much enthusiasm.   Which shows it can and is being done.

So prepare your mind.   Get motivated.   Commit yourself to a hard day's work. It's like diving into an ice-cold sea.   Hesitate and you're lost but once you're in, there's nothing more exhilarating.   Then do it again and again, day in and day out because it's good for you and your mental health. For you! Not some mystical stranger.

You're going to gain so do it for yourself.

SYMPTOM # 16
GUILT

You're feeling guilty because you're not as productive as you once were. What do you expect?   You're handicapped. We're not all like Sir Winston Churchill who rose to tremendous heights through determination and grit. And whose work was made so many times more difficult because of his handicap.

Guilt and depression go together like Wimbledon and strawberries. You wouldn't expect a sightless person to see or someone with defective hearing to heed. So why demand so much of yourself? Why demand what you can't produce. You're sick? Because depression is an illness. A major one according to the UN World Health Organisation. In any one year period, the American National Institute of Mental Health estimates that about 18,8 million American adults suffer from a depressive illness.   That's about 9,5 percent of the population and that's ignoring teenagers and younger kids. Which is frightening but that's the way depression is going.

Recovery will be more difficult if you lean on yourself too much. I know you've got a job and you rely on your paycheck. And the guys at work don't seem to understand what depression is all about and won't until it hits them. Then they'll know and understand and commiserate. But you don't wish it on them or on anyone so you grit your teeth, clamp your jaws and try to get on with it. But please leave the guilt behind. Even without it, you've got enough on your plate.

SYMPTOM # 17

ANXIETY:

Because anxiety is so closely linked to depression, it is often impossible to tell the symptoms apart. But there is a difference. Anxiety is usually an acute state where every problem is exaggerated. Where the outcome of a situation teeters, in the mind, on the catastrophic. Everything you're about to do will be potentially lethal. You're going to fall in the street and die. Eat and you'll choke. You'll be caught in deadly crossfire during an armed robbery. You'll lock yourself out of your home or fall down the stairs. Something bad will happen to you if you get out of bed. A tsunami. A volcanic eruption. Or just an ordinary Richter 7 earthquake!

So what do you do about it? Regard it as just another symptom of depression. That's not exactly what it is but it matters little. Apply what you do for depression and you'll handle it. But how? You force yourself. Ask yourself if anything bad happened to you yesterday. Or the day before? Lately? Ever? Then tell yourself nothing will happen to you today either. I know it's easy to write about but it's possible. All you need do is to get busy. Figuratively speaking, get out of that bed!

SECTION II:

7   TYPES OF DEPRESSION

For reasons already explained, I won't labour you with chapters of clinical detail.   What I *will* do is quote public domain stuff taken from the Internet, from the United States National Institute of Mental Health documentation. For a start, we'll deal only with three basic depression categories remembering that, like many other illnesses, each can have many different variants.

Firstly we have

<u>Major Depression,</u> controlled by a combination of symptoms which effect your life making it difficult to work, to sleep, to eat and enjoy times once relished.   Generally a very disabling type of depression.

<u>Dysthemia.</u> Like major depression, this is also known as Unipolar depression. Something less severe than major depression but involving long-term chronic symptoms that, while not disabling, keeps one from "firing on all cylinders".   Many dysthemia sufferers also have major depressive episodes moments in their lives.

<u>Bipolar Disorder</u> also known as manic-depressive illness.   While this state is not as prevalent as other depressions, it is notable because of severely changing

moods with severe highs (manic) and lows (depression). These mood changes can be dramatic but are usually more gradual. When in the depressive cycle, the sufferer can display typical depressive symptoms. In the manic state, the individual may be elated and hyperactive. Mania can cause major problems and embarrassment. No major business or personal decisions involving marriage, divorce, job changes, etc should be taken when in the manic state because judgement may be disturbed. Above all, left untreated, mania can deteriorate to a state of psychosis. So be sure to seek professional help.

8   WHAT CAUSES DEPRESSION?

This is a difficult one because no-one really knows.   But there is evidence that depression can be genetic.   This is truer in bi-polar depression but major depression can also follow the generations trail and is often associated with changes in brain function. Pessimists with low self-esteem, especially those who cannot take too much heat, may be likely candidates but there are a lot more possible causes. It has been shown that illness can result in mental changes. Hormonal changes, cancer, heart disease, stroke, Parkinson's disease and the like can bring on depression. Sufferers can become apathetic and won't care much about their physical needs.

Apart from things like illness, financial problems, the loss of a dear one, even a difficult relationship, can bring on depression. "Very often," according to the US National Institute of Mental Health, "a combination of genetic, psychological and environmental factors is involved in the onset of a depressive disorder. Later episodes of illness typically are precipitated by only mild stress, or none at all."

9   WHO CAN SUFFER FROM DEPRESSION?

Anyone can be a victim. Men, women, the elderly. Children.

Women seem twice as prone as men. Largely, it is thought, because of hormonal factors. Women also shoulder responsibilities at work and in the home. If single parents, they're responsible for caring and bringing up children as well as sometimes caring for their elderly parents. Also, don't discount menstrual cycle changes, pregnancy, miscarriage and menopause. Again, the US NIMH states, "A recent study showed that in the case of severe premenstrual syndrome (PMS), women with a preexisting vulnerability to PMS experienced relief from mood and physical symptoms when their sex hormones were suppressed. Shortly after the hormones were re-introduced, they again developed symptoms of PMS. Women without a history of PMS reported no effects of the hormonal manipulation."

The NIMH continues. "Many women are particularly vulnerable after the birth of a baby. The hormonal and physical changes, as well as the added responsibility of a new life, can be factors that lead to postpartum depression in some women. While transient 'blues' are common in new mothers, a full-blown depressive episode is not a normal occurrence and requires active intervention. Treatment by a sympathetic physician and the family's emotional support for the new mother are prime considerations in aiding her to recover her physical and mental well-being and her ability to care for and enjoy the infant."

Men are less likely to suffer from depression and are less likely to admit to depression although statistics show that the suicide rate in men is four times that of women. Although more women attempt it, men often hide their depression by using alcohol, drugs or by becoming workaholics. In men, depression often manifests as irritability, anger or being discouraged. Consequently, depression may be difficult to recognise which is further exacerbated by the male's relative unwillingness – compared to females - to get help. Men should realise and accept that depression is a real illness that requires treatment.

In the elderly, It is incorrectly accepted that depression is a natural state. What nonsense! When depression occurs, and when it goes untreated, it causes great suffering for the individual and the family. The sufferer's symptoms are usually considered physical and are often missed. But doctors are now learning to recognise depression in the elderly which isn't easy because some symptoms of depression may be the result of an existing illness, or the side effects of medication being taken for it.

No matter what, elderly patients can be helped over their depression by correct treatment. Also, late-life depression can be treated with psychotherapy.

Depression in children is now taken very seriously. Being a topic that must be emphasised, I quote again, at length, from NIMH publication No.00-3561.

"The depressed child may pretend to be sick, refuse to go to school, cling to a parent, or worry that the parent may die. Older children may sulk, get into trouble at school, be negative, grouchy and feel misunderstood. Because normal behaviors vary from one childhood stage to another, it can be difficult to tell whether a child is just going through a temporary 'phase' or is suffering from depression. Sometimes the parents become worried about how the child's behavior has changed or a teacher mentions that 'your child doesn't seem to be himself.' In such a case, if a visit to the child's pediatrician rules out physical symptoms, the doctor will probably suggest that the child be evaluated, preferably by a psychiatrist who specialises in the treatment of children. If treatment is needed, the doctor may suggest that another therapist, usually a social worker or a psychologist, provide therapy while the psychiatrist will oversee medication if it is needed. Parents should not be afraid to ask questions: What are the therapist's qualifications? What kind of therapy will the child have? Will the family, as a whole, participate in therapy? Will the child's therapy include an anti-depressant?   If so, what might the side effects be?"

10
SYMPTOMS OF BI-POLAR DISORDER (MANIC-DEPRESSION)

Exaggerated irritability

Excessive elation coupled with constant talking.

Heightened energy levels.

Impaired judgement.

Reduced need for sleep coupled with grandiose notions.

Heightened sexual desire.

Overactive mind.

Incorrect social behaviour.

11
TYPES OF ANXIETY DISORDERS

While anxiety is a normal natural reaction to stress, it has it's own uses and advantages. It helps you over tense moments like studying for examinations, job interviews, facing emergencies, business problems, having to make a speech; all normal, everyday ups and downs. Anxiety helps you cope with stress and tension and only becomes a problem when it develops into irrational fear of the daily snags that mark our lives. In other words, when anxiety is so out of control that it affects our day to day existence and becomes disabling.

Effective treatment for anxiety disorders is available and new treatments are being developed all the time to help anxiety sufferers lead full enjoyable and healthy lives.

Again, as detailed by the US National Institute of Mental Health (NIMH) part of the US National Institute of Health (NIH), a component of the US Department of Health and Human Services, in their information sheet entitled "Facts About Anxiety Disorders" publication No. OM-99 4152 printed January 1999 and upgraded 04.09.2004, there are five major types of anxiety disorder.

General anxiety disorder (GAD)
Obsessive compulsive disorder (OCD)
Panic disorder.
Post traumatic stress disorder (PTSD)
Social phobia (or social anxiety disorder)

We'll now discuss them briefly.

General Anxiety Disorder (GAD)

GAD is the name for constant, exaggerated worrisome thoughts and tension about everyday routine life events and activities which last for at least six months.

People with this disorder usually expect the worst; they worry excessively about money, health, family or work even when there are no signs of trouble. The NIMH estimates that about 4 million Americans aged between 18 and 54 have GAD during any given year.

Obsessive Compulsive Disorder (OCD)

This involves repeated unwanted thoughts or compulsions that seem impossible to stop or control. OCD can occur in childhood, adolescence and adulthood but usually first manifests in the teen years or early adulthood.

Panic Disorder

Repeated symptoms of intense fear of having a spontaneous panic attack that can strike often and without warning. Physical symptoms include chest pain, heart palpitations, shortness of breath, dizziness, abdominal distress, feelings of unreality and fear of dying.

Post-Traumatic Stress Disorder

Persistent symptoms that occur after experiencing or witnessing some traumatic event. Such as rape or other criminal assault, war, child abuse, natural or human-caused disasters. The list is endless. Resultant nightmares, flashbacks, emotional numbness, depression, anger, irritability or distraction and being easily startled are common. Note that the family members of victims can also develop this disorder.

Social Phobia (or Social Anxiety Disorder)

Two major types of this phobia are social phobia and specific phobia. People with *social* phobia have an overwhelming and disabling fear of scrutiny, embarrassment, or humiliation in social situations which leads to avoidance of many potentially pleasurable and meaningful activities. People with *specific* phobia experience extreme disabling and irrational fear of something that poses little or no actual danger; the fear leads to avoidance of objects or situations and can cause people to limit their lives unnecessarily.

SOME SYMPTOMS OF ANXIETY DISORDERS

Generalised Anxiety Disorder (GAD)
Inability to relax.
Insomnia.

Fatigue, trembling, muscular tension, headaches, irritability or hot flushes.

Obsessive Compulsive Disorder (OCD)

* Obsessed with a continual need to do things. e.g. checking things over and over or continually washing the hands or counting things.

* Being continually harassed by unwelcome thoughts or images

Note: Symptoms are only diagnosed as OCD if they last for at least an hour a day.

* Include certain symptoms of GAD.

Panic Disorder

* Repeated episodes of intense fear.

* Chest pain, heart palpitations, shortness of breath.

* Dizziness, abdominal pain or discomfort, fear of death, feelings of unreality.

* Include certain symptoms of GAD.

Post Traumatic Stress Disorder (PTSD)

* Symptoms that persist after experiencing trauma.

* Depression.

* Nightmares.

* Jitteriness.

* Anger and being short tempered.

* Numbed emotions.

Note: Family members can also experience PTSD.

* Include certain symptoms of GAD.

Social Phobia [or Social Anxiety Disorder]

* An overwhelming fear of being scrutinised.

* Of being humiliated or embarrassed in public.

* Inability to write or sign one's name in public.

Can lead to avoiding certain pleasant social situations like dining out.

* Include certain symptoms of GAD.

Social Phobia also includes *Specific* Phobia

* Disabling, irrational fear of things which are not dangerous.

* Leads to deliberate avoidance of situations.

Unnecessary avoidance of situations limits pleasures of life like dining out, flying, travel.

*Include certain symptoms of GAD.

CAN YOU SUFFER ANXIETY TOGETHER WITH OTHER MENTAL & PHYSICAL DISORDERS?

Yes! Anxiety usually goes hand in glove with depression and its symptoms. As well as other major illnesses. Obviously the accompanying disorder/s should be treated as well as the anxiety. But it is important to note that a complete medical examination is necessary before anxiety treatment is prescribed as other possible physical causes could cause or relate to the actual symptoms being investigated.

In other words, <u>always see your medical practitioner.</u>

ARE TREATMENTS FOR ANXIETY ORDERS EFFECTIVE?

Yes! And some of the treatments for Depression have also been found to be very effective for treating Anxiety disorders. In many cases, treatment combines medication and psychotherapy. The newest antidepressant drugs known as SSRIs (Selective Serotonin Reuptake Inhibitors) while other anti-anxiety drugs include benzodiazepines and beta-blockers are available. If any one drug does not help, others are usually tried until satisfactory relief is attained. New drugs are continually being developed for the treatment of anxiety.

Two effective forms of psychotherapy have been clinically proven. Behavioural therapy and cognitive-behavioural therapy. Behavioural therapy concentrates on changing certain specific behaviours and employs certain techniques to stop unwanted actions while cognitive-behavioural therapy seeks to teach patients how to change their thought patterns with the view to getting them to a state where they can react differently to what is generating their anxiety.

SECTION III:

12

DEALING WITH CANCER.

Up to now, I've concentrated on how to beat depression. One's *attitude* to cancer should follow the same general pattern. Although it presents itself clinically as something completely different (which it obviously is), cancer, first and foremost, in *all* it's forms and there are many, may be life threatening but not always fatal. It depends largely on early detection. The earlier the greater the chance of recovery. Because of the tremendous advancement in medical science and the astonishing way those achievements have percolated through to the population via a dynamic medical profession, cancer can be cured.

My personal philosophy and attitude towards cancer is naturally influenced by the cancers to which I have been subjected. One has got to be philosophical about all cancers because, besides seeking medical help, there's nothing much else one can do about it beforehand. Unless you're into antioxidants and things, which, in my very humble opinion, don't amount to much.

Firstly, admit that you're a sufferer because cancer usually happens to someone else. Until it gets you! Then act immediately.

You can fight cancer by being positive. I told myself that I would win through, that my cancer would not beat or overpower me. I never doubted that for a moment, not for one moment in fourteen years and I'm still around. Still around and active although, for a while, depression robbed me of some of my zest. But now I'm out and about. I still swim in the ocean and the water's still wonderfully cold and I still enjoy the company of my beach buddies.

Thank You, God. Thank you my wonderful doctors. I thank that wonderful team for their expertise, their kindness, empathy and amazing proficiency.

What has my story to do with anyone but the writer? You must have asked the question so I'll answer. I suppose I've told my story hoping that others might relate to it. Even if only to an attitude, a phrase or an expression which sometimes describes everything.

Because of my cancer and beyond the physical and emotional strain I've endured, I still strongly believe in my faith and the power of even the depression tarnished mind. Much has been said about the power of positive thinking. The expression is now a cliché but it has a sound foundation of truth. I've always maintained that the mind is more than flesh, that mental exertion is greater than the physical, that the body is nothing without the mind and that the mind can exist beyond the body. When it becomes the soul.

Mindset in matters of mortality is crucial to survival. I've seen extremely ill patients stay alive for an important event and then quickly succumb. I have seen retired people waste away through boredom. That's why mental stimulation is life blood to the body, nectar for the soul. Mental stimulation does not necessarily have to do with intellect. As Albert Einstein said. "We should take care not to make the intellect our God. It has, of course, powerful muscles, but no personality." And of our Creator he also said, "God is subtle but he is not malicious."

Where does that place us when fighting cancer? When struggling with mortality? When the fear abates, what is left for us? Certainly a zest for and the love of life itself. And a determined resolve that it not be cut short. Our end must come. That is what we all, friend and foe alike, share. When our lifetime nears it's end, when the time arrives, we must humbly accept finality. Strangely, that is how depression by its constant reference to mortality, prepares us. When depressed, we think of death as an escape so when we have regained normality, death's prospect isn't shrouded too tightly by fear. Because we depressants have been there before. Because it has to do with the mind, approach your fight   with a measure of levity because it suggests confidence and faith.

.Above all, keep on with your life. It's too precious to cast away. Never live your cancer every minute of every day. Get and stay occupied. Stop thinking of your illness as if it belongs to you alone, that it is something only you endure. Cherish what you have, cherish the life you live, cherish your family. Don't yearn for what you haven't got. Above all, believe. In God Almighty. The Creator of Heaven and Earth. Who does and has done wondrous things. Pray to Him daily. Thank Him daily. Pray for His kindness and tell Him how grateful you are for the blessings He has heaped on you.

Keep reading, learning, discovering. Build on your knowledge. The mind is paramount because that's where it all starts. And ends.

Use the time you have left. Gain from what the Lord has given you. Appreciate every sight you see, every thought, every sensation you experience. Enjoy life because it is so short and can be so good.

13

A SUMMATION

Analyse the depressive symptoms and accept that you're depressed. Then get medical advice. Your doctor will know if you're depressed. Don't complicate your problem by denial. Remember, depression isn't a weakness. You're ill and need treatment. Admit your depression to yourself and those close to you.

Medication is essential. So choose the people you'd best like to help you. Understand, they may have to chop and change the medication until they find what best suits you. It'll take a while for the "right stuff" to start working and it is essential that you only take medication under supervision. So listen to your practitioner and follow his instructions.

Eating. Eat healthy food and don't smoke. Exercise. Walking is fine. Choose your distance and pace then build it up gradually. Soon you'll feel better. Your eating will improve and you'll sleep soundly. Get into it gradually and stay with it even after you've beaten depression.

Be with people! This cannot be stressed enough. Depression thrives on loneliness. Depression exaggerates negative thoughts, keeps you harping on the bad without recognising the good. There's good and bad in everything so, if you gain nothing else from this book, make a point of being with people! Make new friends. Get involved. Whatever you do, avoid loneliness.

Try **laughter.** It may not be the easiest thing to do but it's worth a try. Smile or laugh. If you can't smile, grin. If you can't laugh, chuckle. Remember, it is easier to smile than to scowl. It's easier to be nice than to be nasty. Let your personality shine through your laughter.

Be occupied. This is the true secret. Depression doesn't stand a chance against an occupied mind. The trick is to stay occupied. So get there and stay there.

Be positive. You are what you think so you'll be what you think. Instead of giving it up, give it a try.

Routine. It is essential to develop a routine. Routine will help you along. You'll be on the right path without having to think about it.

Do. If anything needs doing, do it! Try. Procrastinate now! Do it because it'll prove that even though you're depressed, you're not useless. That you're as good as you've always been. Doing will re-condition your mind.

Plan. Everything starts in the mind so get into the habit of planning your day.

Sleep and rest. Get your full quota every night.

Read instead of watching television. Imagine scenes, faces and characters. Exercise your mind.

Prayer works for everyone. Especially those private, personal prayers. Bare your mind to your Creator and ask for His help. You'll get it. So believe.

Personal hygiene. Be strict with yourself.

Anxious?   Whatever you do for depression will also help your anxiety. Treat both ailments as one. But see your doctor. He'll sort you out.

Reduced quality of life.   Make do with what you have left.

THAT'S IT. THANK YOU FOR READING THIS
LITTLE BOOK.

www.ingramcontent.com/pod-product-compliance
Lightning Source LLC
Chambersburg PA
CBHW031243280526
45784CB00004B/1702